FAST WEIGHT LOSS
TRICKS
THAT WORK

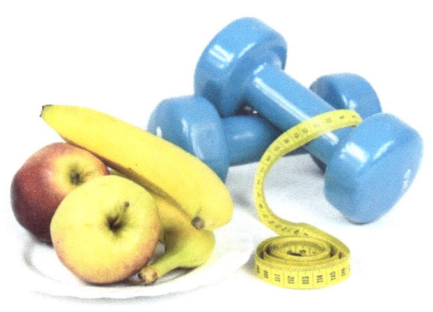

INCREDIBLY EASY WAYS TO LOSE WEIGHT

Table of Contents

Introduction

Healthy diet is one of the most important things that can be done for losing weight. A diet may also affect your health and body resistance problems. It is very important to decide a perfect and healthy diet.

To decide a healthy diet and perfect diet you just need common sense and changes in regular food habits. You can also get free weight loss programs and weight loss plans in the market. To decrease your weight you have to select right foods for your diet plan. Include the foods which are rich in nutrients, minerals and vitamins. Each food has its own nutritional values.

For example some foods have good content of vitamins and some have more content of anti oxidants in it. Some fruits and vegetables are rich in fiber content which can also be included in your regular diet.

You can include all types of foods in your diet so that you may not suffer from nutritional deficiencies. You should also add meat, fish for essential fatty acids. It is better to eat small meals than large meals. You should constantly intake the food so that you can sustain the metabolism. By this your fat will be burned. You have to choose the diet such that you should not feel hungry frequently. For this you have to take some fruits or vegetables as snacks.

For losing weight you have to choose a perfect nutritional plan. Everyone wants to get rid of at least five to ten pounds. Before you start your plan you have to challenge yourself that you will decrease your weight which builds your confidence levels.

Do not plan a diet which is very hard to implement. Do not add the foods which you hate to eat. Plan your diet which is simple, healthy. Add the foods which are liked by you. Add only the foods which low fat content.

You should always have a positive motivating factor which helps your interest in decreasing weight. If you cannot plan a perfect diet then the total fault and responsibility is yours. If you are not able to plan perfect and healthier diet then ask the persons who have already lost their weight by diets or else you can consult a nutritional expert or doctor.

Your diet should not contain the foods that are rich in fats and calories by which you can lead to harmful diseases like high blood pressure, heart attacks and many more.

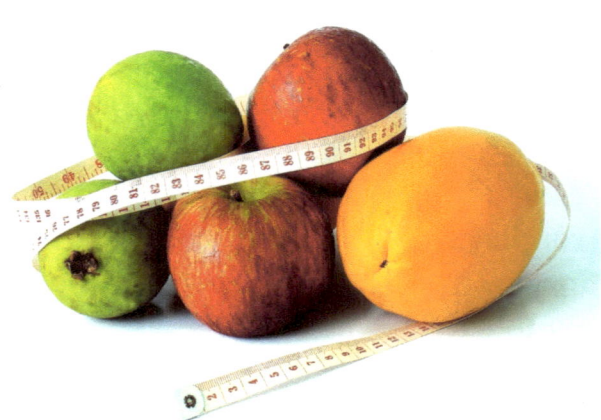

I Need to Lose Weight Fast!

The need to lose weight can be so strong that it drives most people to even hurt themselves in the process, by starving themselves and taking so-called diet pills which do nothing but mess up the metabolism or make the user quite sick. You might not even lose the weight but end up getting hospitalized instead.

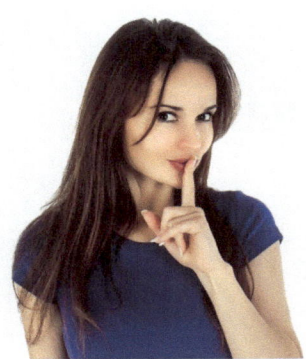

You can lose weight fast, if you follow these tips:

Watch your liquid intake. Makes sure you drink a lot of water, about 8 glasses of water every day. Abstain from drinks such as carbonated beverages, artificial fruit juices - in fact, stay a way from any sweet drink.

Steer clear from alcoholic drinks. Why? Because they are packed with sugar and will only lead to what is known as empty calories - these are calories that are bad for the body and have no nutritional benefit whatsoever.

You will soon be on your way to losing weight quickly and safely when you switch sweet drinks with water.

This might not sound like music to the ears for many people, but learn to exercise all the time.

Weight loss experts will always advice that you should include exercises to your plans for losing weight - this way, you are sure of shedding a couple of pounds safely and effectively.

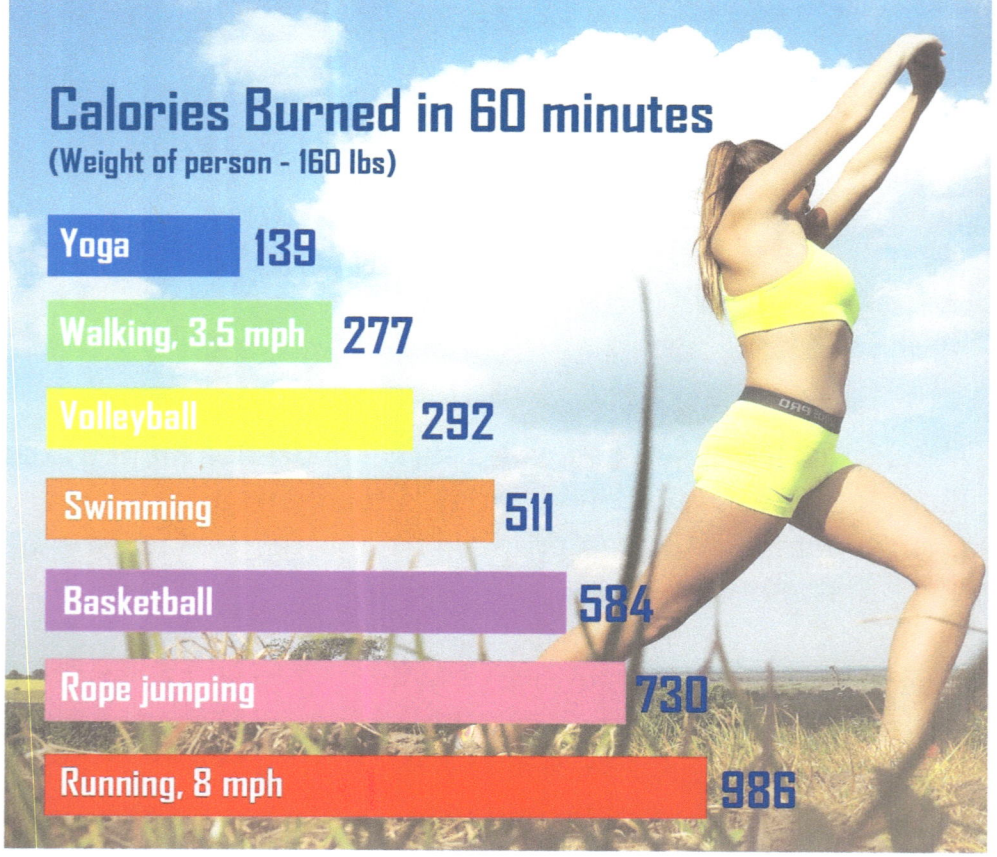

Calories Burned in 60 minutes
(Weight of person - 160 lbs)

Exercise	Calories
Yoga	139
Walking, 3.5 mph	277
Volleyball	292
Swimming	511
Basketball	584
Rope jumping	730
Running, 8 mph	986

You can start your exercise regimen by taking long walks, and as you go on, you can partake in a more rigorous routine.

If you do not like the regular exercise routine, you can spice it up by playing games that will keep your heart rate up, games such as: basketball, tennis, volleyball, etc. Playing these games will keep you sweating and help you burn calories.

Love to eat huh? In order to loose weight fast, you need to learn how to cut down your regular food portions. You should eat food until you no longer feel the hunger pangs and not until you feel stuffed. The most effective way to lose weight and keep it off is to consume less calories and too much fatty foods.

If you must use supplements to boost your metabolism, you should ensure that the supplements are 100 percent natural and safe. Many weight loss pills are being sold everywhere, but you really have to be careful as to the type of drugs you ingest. There are some drugs that come highly recommended for losing weight but it is your responsibility to find out the efficacy of these supplements - it is for your own good.

If you really need to lose weight and you can't seem to do it on your own, you can employ the help of a good weight loss program. A weight loss program can help you change your eating habits, help you exercise and also teach you ways of controlling your food portions. A weight loss program does not have to cost you arm or leg, you can select a program that suits your budget perfectly.

Losing weight can lead to a whole of benefits, it can enhance your physical appearance increase your confidence and lead to a healthy body. confidence and lead to a healthy body.

How to Break That Sugar Habit
and
Lose Weight Fast

It's not news that sugar is linked to weight gain and ill health, so reasonably cutting down on sugar will help you health wise.

However, you may be surprised to learn that there's sugar in ketchup, canned vegetables, luncheon meats, bacon, fast-food hamburgers, and even sushi.

Don't be fooled by products that are labeled low fat or diet either, many of them are loaded with sugar to make them taste better.

The main problem with sugar is that most sources (like candy, soft drinks, and desserts) don't provide appreciable amounts of other nutrients, such as vitamins and minerals, and are therefore classified as "empty calories".

Read ingredient labels for hidden sugar!

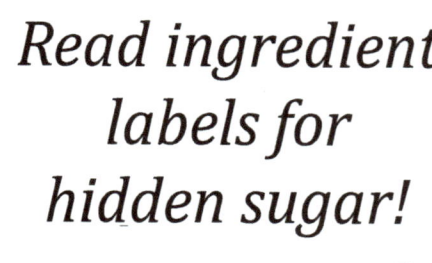
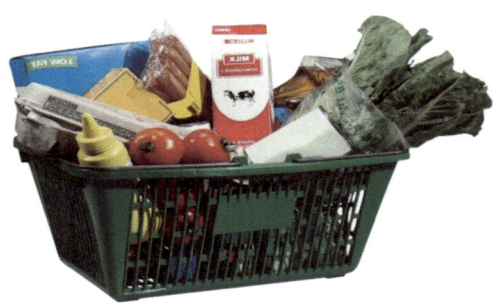

How Much Sugar Is In Your Food?

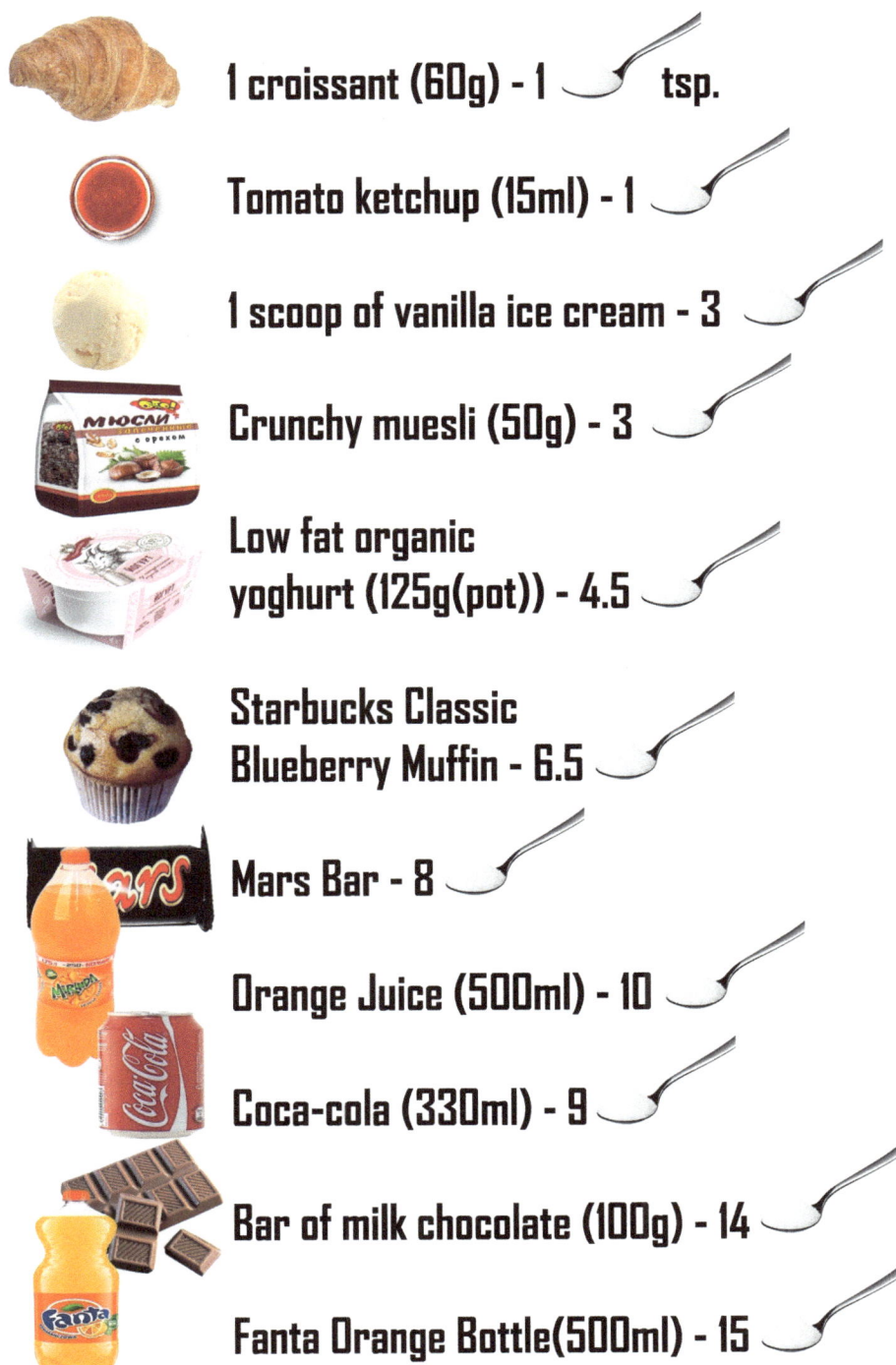

1 croissant (60g) - 1 tsp.

Tomato ketchup (15ml) - 1

1 scoop of vanilla ice cream - 3

Crunchy muesli (50g) - 3

Low fat organic
yoghurt (125g(pot)) - 4.5

Starbucks Classic
Blueberry Muffin - 6.5

Mars Bar - 8

Orange Juice (500ml) - 10

Coca-cola (330ml) - 9

Bar of milk chocolate (100g) - 14

Fanta Orange Bottle(500ml) - 15

So here are a few tips to reduce your consumption of "empty calorie" sweets:

 Satisfy your sweet tooth with fruits, which are good sources of many vitamins and minerals.

 Choose sweets that provide some nutrients, such as ice cream, frozen yogurt, or desserts that contain some fruits and/or nuts. Though the calories and fat may be higher, the extra nutrients make an important contribution to your diet.

 Don't completely deprive yourself of foods you really like because you're more likely to binge to satisfy the need they fulfill and may end up consuming more calories overall. Instead, set reasonable, flexible goals for including sweets in your diet.

 Prepare recipes with half, or two-thirds, of the sugar originally called for.

 Learn to separate physical hunger from emotional hunger. If you eat from emotional hunger (stemming from boredom, stress, or loneliness, for example) you're more likely to overeat low-nutrient foods.

 When you crave something sweet, try a teaspoon or two of jam or preserves on a slice of whole wheat toast, or dip a few strawberries in some honey.

 Reduce the sugar you take in at breakfast by using unsweetened cereal. You can add in some honey.

 Bonus: Don't ever use artificial sweeteners like Splenda, or aspartame, a common ingredient in commercial chewing gum - they are linked to cancer.

Lose Weight Fast by Killing Bad Habits and Making Better Ones

Whether it is biting our finger nails, or leaving the toilet seat up, we all have habits; some good, some not so good.

As a fellow traveler on the journey to health and weight loss, I recognize that many of my weight issues are the result of bad habits. I want to lose weight fast, but how can I lose weight fast with my love for fast food?

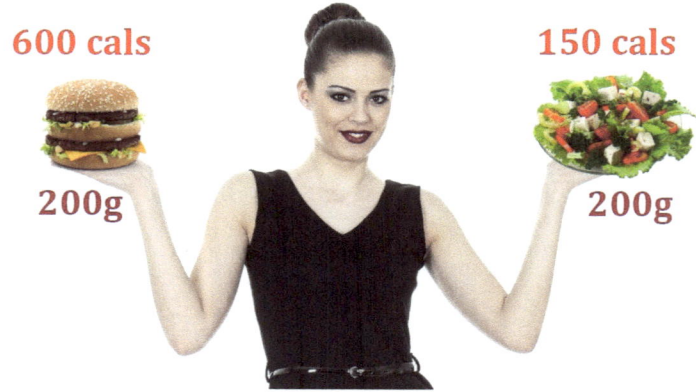

Think about it. Why do I eat that late night snack? Am I actually hungry enough to eat, or have I just "programmed" this to be part of my routine.
This can manifest itself in many different ways, and can be very revealing when you stop and examine things a little more closely, but in what areas could your struggle with weight be connected to bad habits you may have? In what ways could your habits be keeping you from losing weight fast?

As you think about that more closely, we all have have habits that we would like to either form or break.

Hopefully this book can be of help in creating good habits, killing the bad ones, and helping you lose weight the quick and easy way.

 ## *Set An Achievable Goal*

Be positive in your wording. For example, instead of saying, "I will quit snacking at night," say, "I will practice healthy eating habits."

Write your goal down, and perhaps ask someone to help keep you on track.

Be sensible, but also stretch yourself. In other words, don't expect to lose 100lbs by next week, but neither set your goal at only 2lbs per month, when you could potentially lose 2lbs per week.

It might not seem like you're losing weight fast, but 2lbs a week adds up very quickly!

Find Something To Replace Your Bad Habit

This step is very important when you are trying to break a habit.

Many people chew gum when tempted to smoke. This eventually becomes a habit, and replaces the old with the new.

Find your own way of replacing that bad habit with a new, better habit.

Learn Your Triggers

Most likely, you didn't form your habit for no reason. There is usually a "trigger" associated with our habits.

If you're watching TV, you naturally reach for a bag of chips.

Recognize the "common denominators" of your bad habits, and think of possible workarounds.

Be Positive And Remind Yourself Daily Of Your Goals

Even if you mess up, don't lose hope. Be positive, and believe that you CAN break this habit.

Often times when a person over eats once, they assume they might as well binge eat while they have a chance, as soon they will have to start eating healthy again.

Don't do this. This will not only keep you from losing weight fast, it will keep you from losing weight at all! Leving yourself positive reminders can also be a great help.

Leaves notes on the fridge, on your bathroom mirror, or anywhere you see often.

Don't Go At It Alone

John Maxwell once said, "Teamwork makes the dream work."

Things get done more easily and more proficiently with a team effort.

While you can only lose weight yourself, having encouraging people to support you, can make or break your weight loss efforts.

Find someone to share the journey with you, and you will more likely arrive at your destination.

 ### *Write Daily Kudos*

Believe in yourself, that you can achieve your goals. Write them down in the present tense, as if they had already been accomplished.

I have lost weight. I have quit smoking. Let this seep into your subconscious.

Write it every day, ten times a day, for 21 days, and just see what happens!

 ### *Reward Yourself And Be Flexible*

Take small steps to reach your larger goal, but reward yourself at each step along the way.

After all, if you never take that first step, you'll never get anywhere.

If your goal is to lose weight, you don't have to stuff your self silly, but maybe a little extra chocolate will be just what you need!

This will provide both incentive and motivation to continue.

Depending on what you struggle with, it may take several tries for the new habit to take form.

But if you stick with, you'll drop that bad habit in no time! It typically takes about 4 weeks for a new behavior to become routine, or habit, so don't give up!

After all, it did take you more than one day to develop that habit, and it might take you more than one day to break it, but the good news is...you CAN break it!

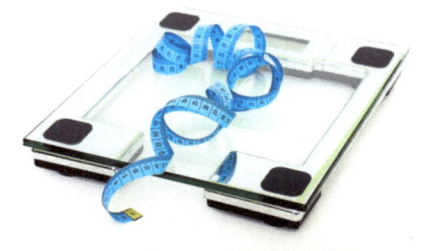

How to Lose Weight Fast
Without Pills

Taking pills to lose weight is never the answer and you know it. Hey, that's why you are here, right?

Stuffing various chemicals in your body and hoping for a miracle can have devastating effects on your health.

But you are not here to read about the side effects, you want to know how to lose weight fast without pills. So let me tell you.

You probably know this one already that exercise is just one alternative. You don't need it to effectively lose weight. Sure, by exercising daily you can lose fat, but only if changing your old eating habits.

If you eat the right foods at the right time, you could even lose weight by sitting at home all day doing nothing. Now, I am not saying you should do that.

What I am trying to tell you here is that exercise is good for you (duh) and you should do it whenever possible.

Also, if combining exercise with healthy eating habits, you could do even better - lose all your excessive weight faster.

I think by now you already know, what I mean by healthy eating habits. That's right, a diet. "But a diet is even worse, I have to eat only the foods I hate and starve myself..."

This is what most people associate with a diet and why they avoid it at all cost. And who can blame them? Would you starve yourself and eat only the foods you hate?

You wouldn't probably finish this diet anyway and even if you did, by returning to the old eating habits the weight would return as well. But you should know that not every diet is this bad.

There are some fast and balanced weight loss diets that don't force you to starve and are really enjoyable.

So, if you would ask me how to lose weight fast without pills, my answer would be this kind of diet.

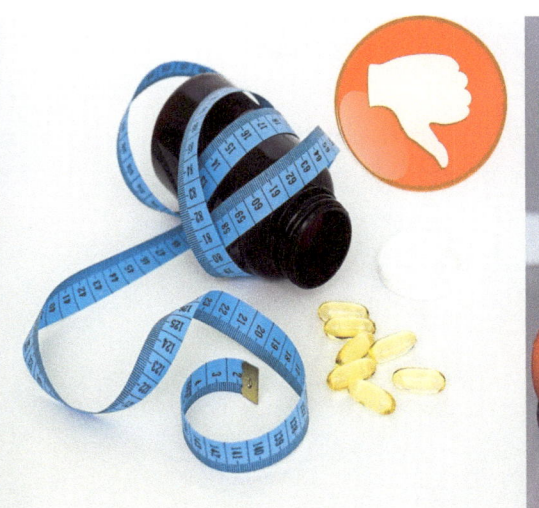 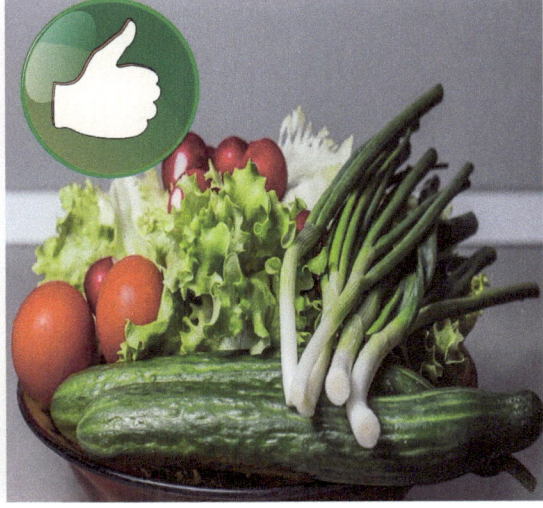

Is Your Diet A Fad Diet -
How Do I Lose Weight Fast?

A lot of diets get the reputation of being a fad diet. This is not necessarily true. Most diets when you first start them could be considered a fad diet because of all the carbs they take out of your plan so that they can achieve the original weight loss promise.

The truth is that after the first couple of weeks they start adding good carbs back into the diet. They only restrict it so much to start with because they know that a lot of people don't like to exercise and would refuse to start or try their diet plan if it includes a lot or sometimes even just a small amount of exercise.

The problem comes in because they restrict the diet so much that people can't maintain it so they quit and it becomes just one more failed diet attempt.

What originally got many overweight people in trouble is that they are unable to control themselves. They find that complete freedom leads to bad choices. That's why diets like this work well for short periods of time.

Dieters like to feel that they've regained control over their eating habits.

However even though you are certain to lose weight on these plans it's easy to fall off the wagon because they are so strict.

Because these diets start out by making a very strict and planned eating portions they get the reputation and must be regarded as, at least in part, a fad diet.

This takes nothing away from the diets that advocate smaller portions of healthy foods spread out over the day combined with 20 to 30 minutes of exercise.

Once somebody get's started on this kind of diet and exercise plan they find it's very easy to maintain. The problem comes in when you mention exercise a lot of people run the other way. They don't even bother trying.

The plain truth is that no matter what diet and exercise program you choose, if you consume more than you burn you will gain weight. If you burn more than you consume you will lose weight. There is no way around this. It works the same way for everybody.

While you can lose weight with diet alone you probably will not be able to maintain the weight loss.

The best way is with a combination of diet and exercise. It develops good habits that make it easy to lose weight fast and keep it off.

My body's metabolizm burns 1800 calories per day

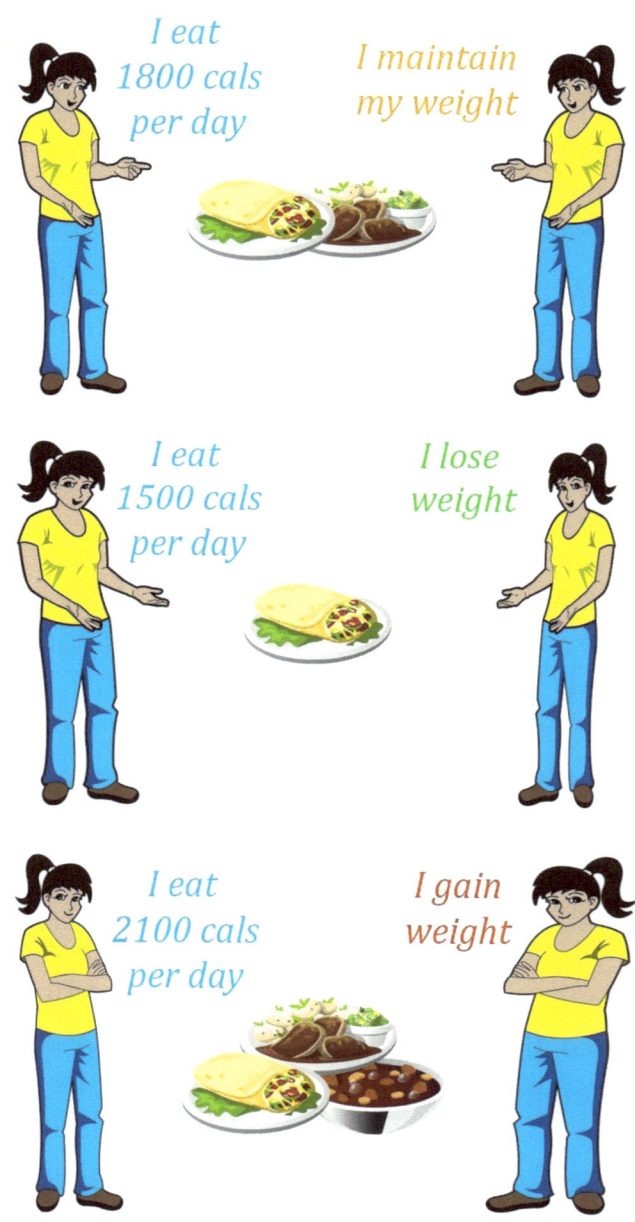

I eat 1800 cals per day

I maintain my weight

I eat 1500 cals per day

I lose weight

I eat 2100 cals per day

I gain weight

Lose Weight Fast -
Why Childhood Obesity Is Increasing

In the United States today, one of every three children is obese. This is the major health issue in that country.

Obesity, especially in people so young, leads to early onset Diabetes, strokes and heart attacks, even in the adolescent years. It may be linked to some cancers.

There are two reasons for this health issue, poor eating habits and lack of exercise.

Your child cannot lose weight fast until both of these deficiencies are corrected. However, that is harder than you think, because most of us crave unhealthy meals.

We eat processed foods which are loaded with artificial colors, sugars and salt. Readymade dinners, breakfasts and lunches fill the freezer sections and shelves of most grocery stores as well as calorie dense deserts, snacks and concentrated fruit juices.

Look at your grocery store, how much of it contains fresh produce, dairy and meat sections, in comparison to processed, canned and frozen foods?

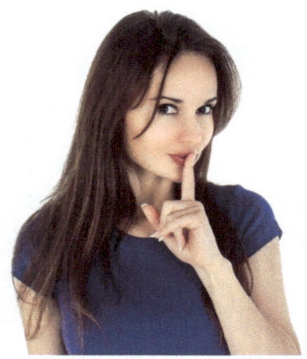

Seek out healthy versions high-calorie foods which taste as good

Unhealthy foods are everywhere because they taste better and more convenient.

There is hardly a store you walk into today which does not have candy and snacks near the checkout counter, including department stores, home improvement stores, even fabric stores and pet stores.

There is a portion of fresh meats, dairy products and eggs contain certain amounts of chemicals fed to animals so they can produce more, grow faster, or stay healthier.

These, according to recent studies, stimulate fat cell growth. Even plants can be injected with chemicals, rubbed with waxes, and given added colors.

They can be picked before they are fully developed and then artificially ripened with gases on the way to market reducing their nutritional value.

People say they can't afford organic foods and locally grown produce and meats. However, health is your most valuable possession so hold it tight and never let it go.

Furthermore, our kids are becoming sedentary, physical education programs have been shortened or cut, computer games and TV have taken the place of physical activities.

Luckily, the newer games get kids active and moving. Still, in the 1960's kids watched an average of 5 hours of TV a week. Today, many watch that much a day.

Good habits start young. If you want your child to lose weight fast, be the parent with the touch love attitude. Stop buying the wrong foods, pack their lunches, talk to them about the importance of good eating habits and make exercise a part of their daily routine.

Finally, kids imitate mom and dad, so follow your own advice. Exercise with them, and share healthy meals together.

You may discover the house is a happier place, everyone sleeps better and doctor visits will be less often. You may even discover that you lose weight fast as well.

Best Healthy Alternatives to Unhealthy Foods

BREAD	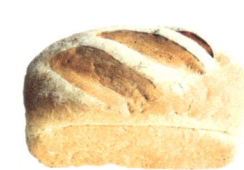	**Sprouted grain breads** **Rye Bread** **Oopsie Bread** **Corn Tortillas**
PASTA	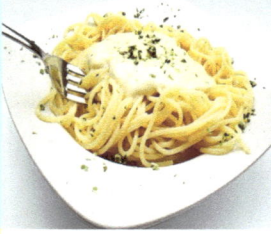	**Zucchini** **Soba Noodles** **Shirataki Noodles** **Brown Rice Pasta**
PORK SAUSAGE	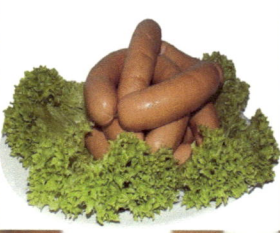	**Turkey Sausage** **Chicken Sausage**
WHOLE MILK	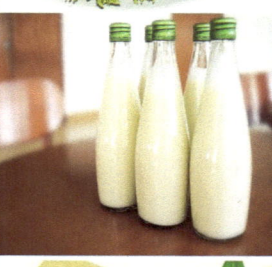	**Non-fat Milk** **Soy Milk** **Coconut Milk** **Rice Milk** **Almond Milk**
BUTTER	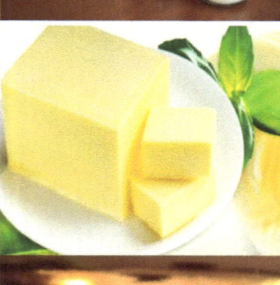	**Avocados** **Greek Yogurt** **Applesauce** **Pumpkin Puree**
SUGARY CEREAL	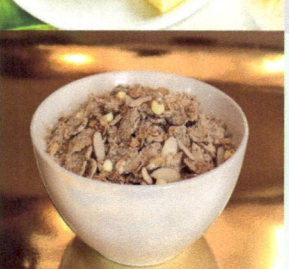	**Porridge** **Quinoa**

CHIPS	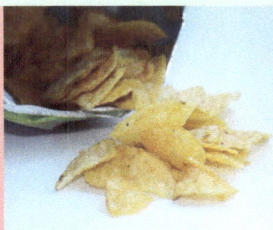	**Homemade Veggie Chips Popcorn Kale chips**
SUGARY DRINKS	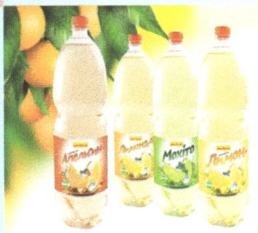	**Homemade Juices Coconut Water Iced Tea Mineral Water**
ICE CREAM	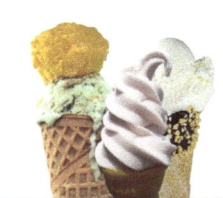	**Frozen Banana Ice Cream Avocado Ice Cream Greek Frozen Yogurt Ice Cream**
CANDY	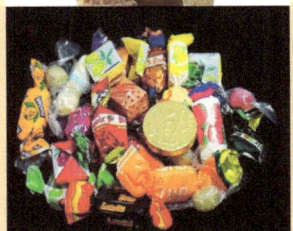	**Dried Fruit Sugar-Free Gum Homemade Dark Chocolate**
COOKIES	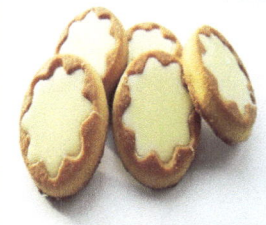	**Homemade Whole Wheat Cookies Pumpkin Chip Cookies**
CROUTONS	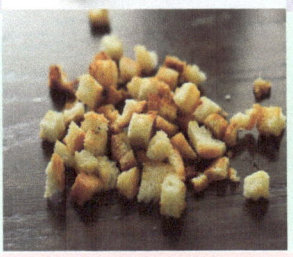	**Roasted Almonds Roasted Chickpeas Pumpkin Seeds**

Here's How to Lose Weight Fast in a Safe and Harmless Way

If you want to lose weight fast then what you need to realize is that it is something that can be very difficult to accomplish, and the fact of the matter is that with some of these fast weight loss methods the results are only short-term instead of long- lasting.

The problem that people have when they gain weight is the fact that they don't have the discipline to stick to a diet or exercise good eating habits.

The first thing you should be doing to help yourself burn fat is getting more vegetables and fruits into the meals that you are eating every day.

You need to discontinue eating foods that are high in fat, and by this I mean all of your comfort foods that are especially sweet that you love to eat at some point during the day.

That's right, you have to stop eating these foods, and if you aren't exercising often then you need to start doing something about that.

For instance, you can start walking on a daily basis, and honestly you need to make it a habit to start walking on a daily basis.

I love all these methods but the only thing you need to be focused on is eating healthier because it doesn't matter what method you use to get rid of weight, if you don't establish healthier eating habits then you will definitely gain all the weight that you lose right back.

The second tip or method that you can take advantage of to help yourself lose weight is to eat those foods that are specifically helpful in losing weight.

Even though you want to be eating these weight loss foods, you also don't want to forget the fact that you should be following a well balanced diet to help you reach your goal.

A lot of people aren't aware of this but drinking unsweetened green tea before-and-after a meal is a phenomenal way to help yourself lose weight without practically any effort put into it.

Even if you don't like the taste of green tea, there are green tea supplements that have been created to help a person lose weight.

You should also be staying away from beverages that are high in carbs and calories, especially those sodas.

Another tip that I've taken advantage of to help myself lose weight personally, is I've had a friend who is trying to lose weight so we both teamed up and helped each other lose weight fast by using each other's methods.

I also recommend that you start doing muscle building exercises to help yourself burn fat and calories fast. Building muscle is a phenomenal way to increase your metabolic rate so please get started on doing strength training exercises to help you build muscle.

I also recommend that you stay away from those fried and grilled foods, and instead replace those with vegetable soups and fruit salads in your diet.

Remember not to overeat when it comes to your meals, and try to eat six small low calorie meals throughout your day, but remember to have a big breakfast so that you aren't constantly hungry for the next meal.

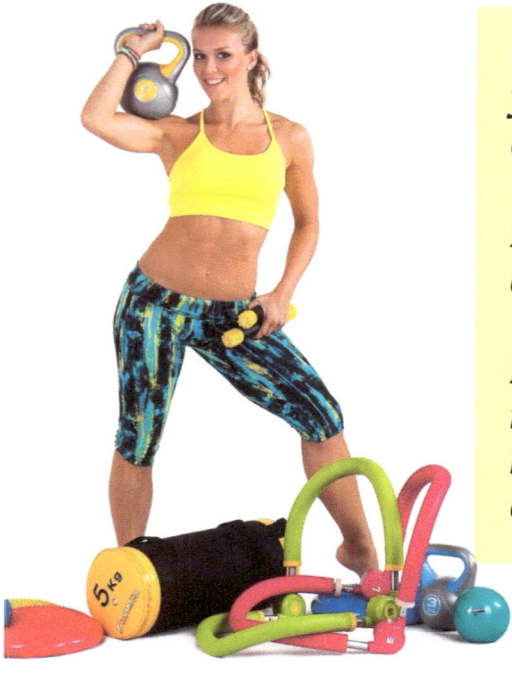

The more muscle mass you have, the more calories you burn at rest.

Muscle tissue eats fat at all hours of the day.

For every pound of muscle gained, the body burns 50 extra calories every day.

Will Yoga Help You Lose Weight Fast?

Yoga offers several health benefits, including improved flexibility, better strength, muscle toning and stress reduction.

It also makes you feel better about your body and reportedly also improves your sense of mental well-being.

However, the question that a lot of people have is whether yoga is really effective as a weight loss workout. If you want to lose weight fast, you probably want to know how well the hard numbers add up.

 ## The Ineffectiveness of Regular Yoga

Unfortunately, most forms of yoga will not help achieve significant weight loss. This is because yoga does not raise your heart rate sufficiently enough and for long enough periods of time to work as a weight loss tool.

On an average, a one-hour long session of yoga will burn about 160 calories for a 150 pound person, whereas a 3 mph walk for the same period of time will burn over 300 calories.

Put simply, the figures don't seem to add up, especially if you are a beginner who is new to fitness and have very little flexibility.

However, if you are already reasonably fit and have good reason to trust your body's current capabilities, yoga can become a means to lose weight fast.

 ## A Powerful Exception

The one form of yoga which can help one lose weight, according to many experts and physical trainers, is known as Vinyasa Yoga.

It involves a series of sun salutations, with varying postures, done without any breaks in-between. The postures are usually quite challenging and become progressively harder over the course of the session.

One is also expected to breathe normally while doing Vinyasa Yoga. Doing this form of yoga will really raise your heart rate and keep it beating fast right through the session.

This is what will eventually help you lose weight!

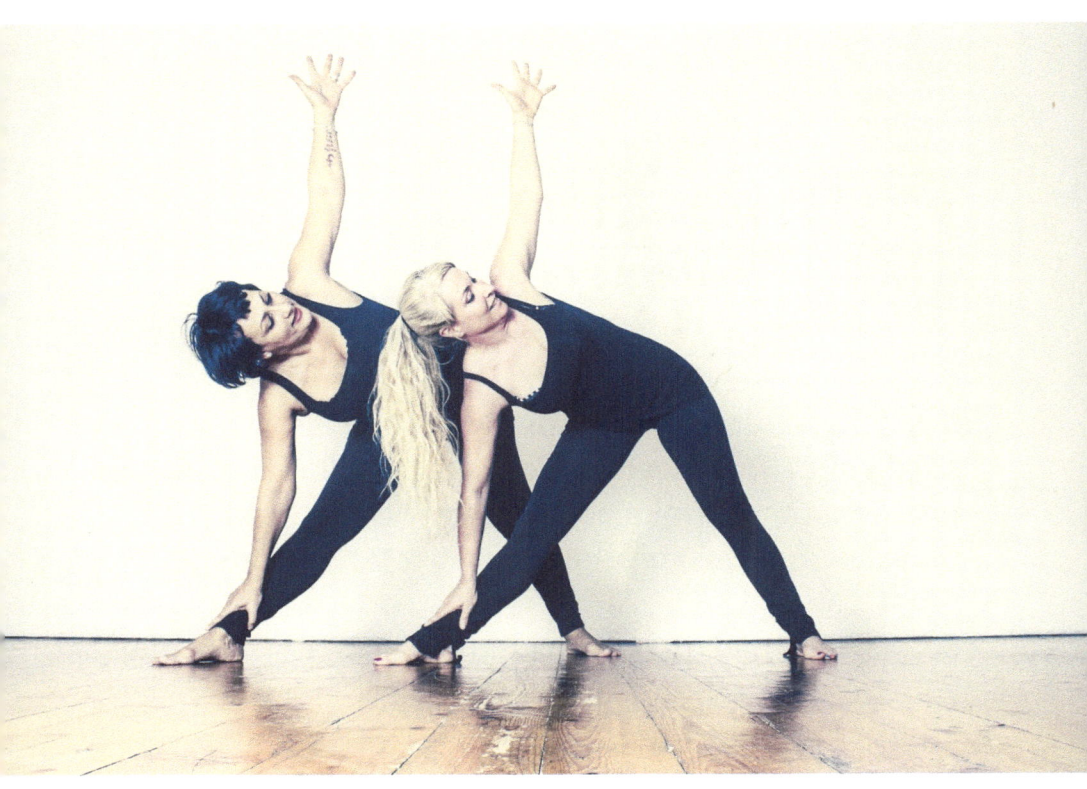

However, practicing any of the forms of Vinyasa Yoga require reasonable levels of fitness, and beginners will need to improve their flexibility and strength before they can get to that level.

The most popular form of Vinyasa Yoga, especially in the west, is known as Power Yoga.

In fact, Power Yoga has now become a very generic te rm used for any strenuous and intense yoga session, a nd different people practice it in completely different ways.

Indirect Weight Loss Benefits of Yoga

Apart from directly burning calories to help you shed your excess weight, yoga also has indirect weight loss benefits. For one, it tones and strengthens your muscles, and this improves your metabolic rate.

So, you will end up burning more calories even while you are at rest. Besides, by reducing your stress levels, improving your sense of well-being and making you connect with and understand your body much better, it also helps you control and regulate your appetite. So, you are less prone to over-eating.

This is why yoga is known to be so effective for people who have already reached a near-perfect weight and want to keep those excess pounds off.

At the end of the day, yoga offers a lot more than just burning calories. It gives you a complete package of health. It will promote good habits and improve your base of strength and flexibility.

So, whatever weight loss exercises you take up, you will be able to do them productively, enjoy them and protect yourself from injuries.

Best Diet Plans
To Lose Weight Fast

Millions of people each day are on a diet of one form or another.

Whether you are just looking to drop a few pounds to fit in a new dress or if you need to drop a lot of weight for health reasons, there are diet plans to lose weight fast available to you.

The key is to choose the right one for you. We have some tips and tricks to help you.

Make sure you are healthy enough for dieting. Check with your physician before you start any new diet or exercise program.

Your health should be your first priority.

If the program is too complicated or cuts out to much then it may be doomed from the start. You have to be able to stick with it for the long term to see the best results and keep the weight off. If not then you may face gaining back any pounds you lost and then some.

Be realistic with your goals. If you expect instant results then you may become discouraged quickly. Chances are that you won't lose twenty pounds in that first week and this is not even healthy if you could. Our weight goes up and down on a daily basis. Know what is normal for you and go from there to judge your success.

Exercise should be part of any program you choose. This helps you burn calories and tone muscles.

Walking a few times a week may be enough for some while others may need a more vigorous workout. This may also help to boost your energy levels. Know your limits and drink plenty of water to keep your body hydrated.

Be sure your daily eating habits include enough calories to meet your energy needs. Some may be tempted to cut calories by far too much and not only can this lead to over eating but it may hinder success and deprive your of essential vitamins and nutrients.

Making good food choices is essential to a successful diet. Some foods can even aide in burning calories and helping to lose pounds.

Choosing foods that are low in calories but high in nutrition can help you meet your body's needs, feel full, and still shed unwanted pounds.

Diet plans to lose weight fast can be very beneficial to many people. Keep in mind that not all diet plans are right for everyone and one of the biggest factors in determining your success may be your ability to follow the plan as recommended and stick with it.

Healthy Eating for a Healthy Weight

BROWN RICE

WHOLE GRAIN

QUINOA

WHHOLE GRAIN PASTA

SWEET POTATO

TUNA

CHICKEN   LENTILS

TURKEY   LEAN BEEF

GREEK YOGURT

COTTAGE CHEESE

OATS

BEANS

STARCH   PROTEIN

EGGS

FISH

TOFU

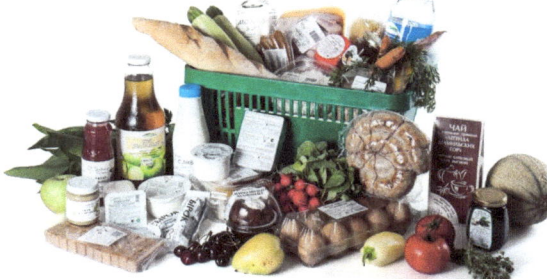

KALE

PEAS

VEGGIE   FATS

FLAX SEED

HEMP SEED

ONIONS

BROCCOLI

CARROTS

CAULIFLOWER

ZUCCHINI

ASPARAGUS   SPINACH

WALNUTS

COCONUT OIL

ALMONDS

AVOCADO

PUMPKIN SEED

Foods
That Will Help You
Lose Weight

So-called "zero-calorie" foods, like asparagus and mushrooms, contain fewer calories than the body uses to break them down.

So what exactly makes them "zero-calorie" foods?

These foods are excellent diet foods because they help you feel full and gain nutrients. Because of their high fiber content, you feel satiated longer than with other foods.

The negative calorie foods control the appetite, boost your metabolism, lower stress and improve your digestion.

Although zero calorie foods may have negligible calories, make no mistake, they still count towards a day's worth of calories.

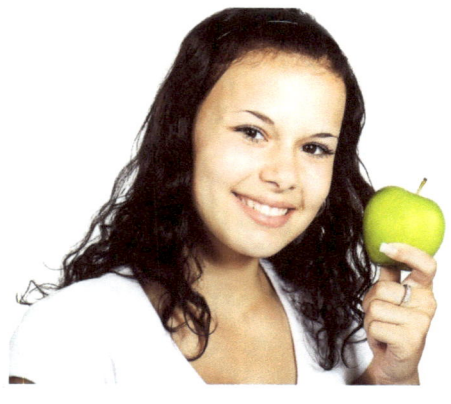

Foods that contain few calories, such as apples or cauliflower provide a small number of calories but still require energy to digest.

Each of These Foods Has Fewer Than 50 Calories per 100g

Cucumber	16	Mushrooms	38
Celery	16	Onions	40
Zucchini	17	Carrots	41
Tomatoes	17	Grapefruit	42
Asparagus	20	Beets	43
Cabbage	25	Blackberries	43
Cauliflower	25	Peaches	45
Pumpkin	26	Plums	46
Turnips	28	Oranges	47
Lemons	29	Kale	49
Watermelon	30	Apples	49
Broccoli	34	Pineapple	50

Fun Ways
to Lose Weight Fast

Slowly but surely, that is the key to losing weight. So take it easy at first and go step by step first by starting off with your eating habits.

Cut down on all your unhealthy fast foods and start eating more healthier foods in your diet such as various vegetables and fruits.

Once you have safely gone through that particular step it then comes time to implement an exercise program to your everyday life.

Again just like losing weight as a whole, take exercising one step at a time if you are not a fan of exercises. Slowly start off with 15-20 minutes of exercising each day and gradually add on the minutes as the days and weeks go by.

Create a series of ten-minute walking trips throughout you day.

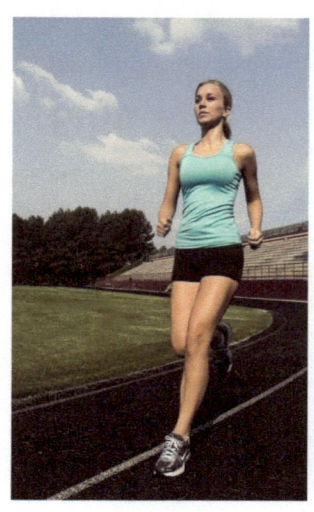

When building muscle mass you tend to lose more calories according to your weight as muscles burn calories at a much higher rate than fat does.

Start lifting more weights in your exercise program to build muscles efficiently and have those extra muscles burn away those unwanted extra calories for the long term.

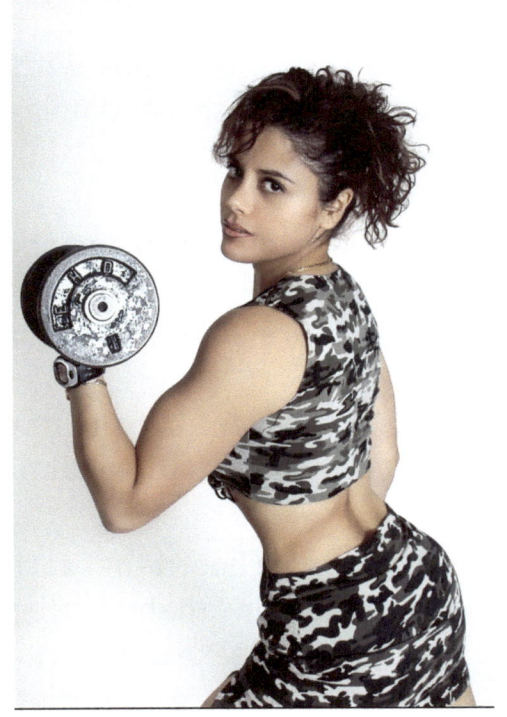

In order to help keep you motivated, always remember it is important to choose exercises and foods that you enjoy because if you do not then you will find that your exercise programs and food are not being effective and you start losing hope.

So choose wisely and have patience when choosing as well!

Do not fool yourself with unachievable goals. This will only demotivate you when you do not successfully achieve it.

So start being honest with yourself and start setting achievable goals and measurable deadlines to achieve them.

Set both long term and short term goals and you will find yourself understanding your weight loss program even more with a clear goal or goals in mind.

This will eventually help with your overall weight loss success in a healthy manner.

If you have heard that carbohydrates are one of the main reasons that people gain weight then it is true. However please do not remove carbohydrates completely from your diet just make sure you reduce your intake of carbohydrates and that is good enough.

The reason for this is because carbohydrates are essential for the body to gain energy. Pastas, rice and bread are some of the things you can cut back on or have a substitute for them so that you will not miss it that much.

For example cut down on the intake of the usual white processed bread and switch to wholemeal bread as there is a slight difference in taste but at the same time benefits you in your weight loss immensely.

Same goes for rice, as you can replace white processed rice for brown rice for better health and fitness as well.

Quit the eating of candies, cakes, cookies or anything with lots of sugar and sweets as it can really blow your mind as to how unhealthy and fattening these snacks really are.

Reduce these snacks by at least 70% or even better if possible cut it out completely from your diet because you do not need them as they do you NO GOOD!

You will even notice gradual weight loss happening without you even doing anything, how amazing is that!

Breakfast is essential. Most of the calories you take in must be consumed earlier in the day so that it can be easily burned off during your performance of everyday activities.

Consume a nice and hearty breakfast to provide a good base for your metabolism to run from for the rest of the day.

Leave some food behind in order to correctly based your food portions on the actual serving size of your food but at the same time make sure you do not completely empty out your plate.

This will really help you in having a good control of the size of the food portion that you are inserting into your body and help in successfully achieving your weight loss goal.

Conclusion

Start using and performing these tips step by step and definitely in due time you will begin to see really huge significant differences in all parts of your body and fitness levels.

Don't believe me?

Start trying it today and see for yoursel!

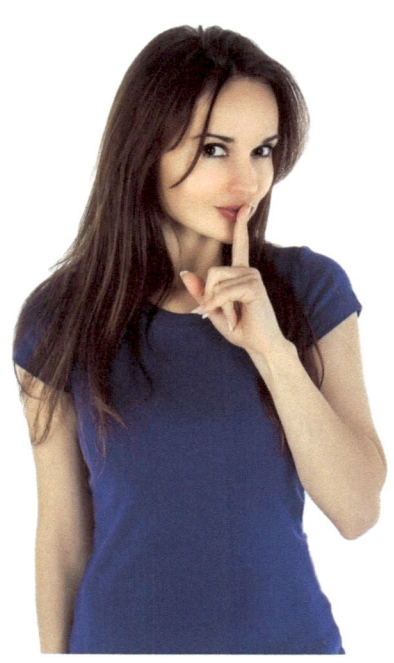

7- DAY MEAL PLAN

	DAY 1	DAY 2
BREAKFAST	½ CUP OATMEAL 1 BOILED EGG 1 SLICE WHOLE WHEAT BREAD 1 TBS PEANUT BUTTER	VEGGIE OMELETTE (2 EGGS WITH 1/3 CUP VEGGIES) 2 SLICES TOAST 1 CUP GREEK YOGURT
SNACK	1 SMALL BANANA	1 CUP FRUIT SALAD
LUNCH	6 OZ CHICKEN BREAST 1 SLICE WHOLE WHEAT BREAD 1 CUP VEGETABLE SALAD	1 CUP OF VEG BASED SOUP 1 SLICE WHOLE WHEAT BREAD ½ CUP TUNA
SNACK	1 CUP BLUEBERRIES	1 GRAPEFRUIT 10 ALMONDS
DINNER	2 OZ TOFU CUTLET 1 CUP BROWN RICE 1 CUP VEGETABLE SALAD	6 OZ LEAN STEAK 1 CUP VEGETABLE SALAD

	DAY 3	DAY 4
BREAKFAST	½ CUP OATMEAL 1 SLICE WHOLE WHEAT BREAD 1 TBS PEANUT BUTTER 1 CUP GREEK YOGURT	2 BOILED EGGS 2 SLICES TOAST 1 CUP FRUIT SALAD
SNACK	1 CUP STRAWBERRIES	1 APPLE 1 SMALL BANANA
LUNCH	6 OZ GRILLED CHICKEN BREAST 1 CUP VEGETABLE SALAD WITH 1 OZ LOW FAT CHEDDAR	1 CUP CHICKEN VEG SOUP 1 SLICE WHOLE WHEAT BREAD 1 CUP TACO SALAD
SNACK	1 CUP COTTAGE CHEESE 1 SMALL ORANGE	10 ALMONDS ½ CUP MIXED BERRIES
DINNER	6 OZ BAKED SALMON 1 CUP VEGETABLE SALAD	2 CUPS STEAMED VEGETABLES 4 OZ CHICKEN BREAST

	DAY 5	DAY 6
BREAKFAST	VEGGIE OMELETTE (2 EGGS WITH 1/3 CUP VEGGIES) 1 SLICE WHOLE WHEAT BREAD 1 TBS PEANUT BUTTER	½ CUP OATMEAL 1 BOILED EGG 1 SLICE TOAST 1 CUP FRUIT SALAD
SNACK	1 CUP MIXED BERRIES	1 CUP COTTAGE CHEESE
LUNCH	1 CUP ZUCCHINI PASTA 2 OZ TOFU CUTLET 1 CUP VEGETABLE SALAD WITH 1 OZ LOW FAT CHEDDAR	6 OZ TURKEY BREAST 1 SLICE WHOLE WHEAT BREAD 1 CUP TACO SALAD
SNACK	1 CUP COTTAGE CHEESE 1 SMALL ORANGE	1 GRAPEFRUIT 20 ALMONDS
DINNER	6 OZ GRILLED CHICKEN 1/2 CUP BLACK BEANS 1 CUP VEGETABLE SALAD	4 OZ BAKED SALMON 1 CUP BROWN RICE 1 CUP VEGETABLE SALAD

DAY 7

BREAKFAST	2 BOILED EGGS 1 SLICE WHOLE WHEAT BREAD 1 TBS PEANUT BUTTER 1 CUP GREEK YOGURT
SNACK	1 CUP FRUIT SALAD
LUNCH	½ CUP TUNA 1 SLICE WHOLE WHEAT BREAD 1 CUP TACO SALAD
SNACK	1 APPLE 10 ALMONDS
DINNER	6 OZ LEAN STEAK 1/2 CUP BROWN RICE 1 CUP VEGETABLE SALAD